Anxiety & Stress

Date:

How I feel this morning:

How I feel this afternoon:

How I feel this evening:

AF429968

Today's Anxiety & Stress Analysis

Causes of my anxiety & stress:	How I can change the causes:
1.	1.
2.	2.
3.	3.
4.	4.
5.	5.
6.	6.
7.	7.
8.	8.
9.	9.
10.	10.
11.	11.
12.	12.
13.	13.

Notes

Anxiety & Stress

Date:

How I feel this morning:

How I feel this afternoon:

How I feel this evening:

Today's Anxiety & Stress Analysis

Causes of my anxiety & stress:

How I can change the causes:

Causes of my anxiety & stress:	How I can change the causes:
1.	1.
2.	2.
3.	3.
4.	4.
5.	5.
6.	6.
7.	7.
8.	8.
9.	9.
10.	10.
11.	11.
12.	12.
13.	13.

Notes

Anxiety & Stress

Date:

How I feel this morning:

How I feel this afternoon:

How I feel this evening:

Today's Anxiety & Stress Analysis

Causes of my anxiety & stress:	How I can change the causes:
1.	1.
2.	2.
3.	3.
4.	4.
5.	5.
6.	6.
7.	7.
8.	8.
9.	9.
10.	10.
11.	11.
12.	12.
13.	13.

Notes

Anxiety & Stress

Date:

How I feel this morning:

How I feel this afternoon:

How I feel this evening:

Today's Anxiety & Stress Analysis

Causes of my anxiety & stress:	How I can change the causes:
1.	1.
2.	2.
3.	3.
4.	4.
5.	5.
6.	6.
7.	7.
8.	8.
9.	9.
10.	10.
11.	11.
12.	12.
13.	13.

Notes

Anxiety & Stress

Date:

How I feel this morning:

How I feel this afternoon:

How I feel this evening:

Today's Anxiety & Stress Analysis

Causes of my anxiety & stress:	How I can change the causes:
1.	1.
2.	2.
3.	3.
4.	4.
5.	5.
6.	6.
7.	7.
8.	8.
9.	9.
10.	10.
11.	11.
12.	12.
13.	13.

Notes

Anxiety & Stress

Date:

How I feel this morning:

How I feel this afternoon:

How I feel this evening:

Today's Anxiety & Stress Analysis

Causes of my anxiety & stress:

How I can change the causes:

1.

1.

2.

2.

3.

3.

4.

4.

5.

5.

6.

6.

7.

7.

8.

8.

9.

9.

10.

10.

11.

11.

12.

12.

13.

13.

Notes

Anxiety & Stress

Date:

How I feel this morning:

How I feel this afternoon:

How I feel this evening:

Today's Anxiety & Stress Analysis

Causes of my anxiety & stress:

How I can change the causes:

Causes of my anxiety & stress:	How I can change the causes:
1.	1.
2.	2.
3.	3.
4.	4.
5.	5.
6.	6.
7.	7.
8.	8.
9.	9.
10.	10.
11.	11.
12.	12.
13.	13.

Notes

Anxiety & Stress

Date:

How I feel this morning:

How I feel this afternoon:

How I feel this evening:

Today's Anxiety & Stress Analysis

Causes of my anxiety & stress:	How I can change the causes:
1.	1.
2.	2.
3.	3.
4.	4.
5.	5.
6.	6.
7.	7.
8.	8.
9.	9.
10.	10.
11.	11.
12.	12.
13.	13.

Notes

Anxiety & Stress

Date:

How I feel this morning:

How I feel this afternoon:

How I feel this evening:

Today's Anxiety & Stress Analysis

Causes of my anxiety & stress:	How I can change the causes:
1.	1.
2.	2.
3.	3.
4.	4.
5.	5.
6.	6.
7.	7.
8.	8.
9.	9.
10.	10.
11.	11.
12.	12.
13.	13.

Notes

Anxiety & Stress

Date:

How I feel this morning:

How I feel this afternoon:

How I feel this evening:

Today's Anxiety & Stress Analysis

Causes of my anxiety & stress:

How I can change the causes:

1.

1.

2.

2.

3.

3.

4.

4.

5.

5.

6.

6.

7.

7.

8.

8.

9.

9.

10.

10.

11.

11.

12.

12.

13.

13.

Notes

Anxiety & Stress

Date:

How I feel this morning:

How I feel this afternoon:

How I feel this evening:

Today's Anxiety & Stress Analysis

Causes of my anxiety & stress:	How I can change the causes:
1.	1.
2.	2.
3.	3.
4.	4.
5.	5.
6.	6.
7.	7.
8.	8.
9.	9.
10.	10.
11.	11.
12.	12.
13.	13.

Notes

Anxiety & Stress

Date:

How I feel this morning:

How I feel this afternoon:

How I feel this evening:

Today's Anxiety & Stress Analysis

Causes of my anxiety & stress:	How I can change the causes:
1.	1.
2.	2.
3.	3.
4.	4.
5.	5.
6.	6.
7.	7.
8.	8.
9.	9.
10.	10.
11.	11.
12.	12.
13.	13.

Notes

Anxiety & Stress

Date:

How I feel this morning:

How I feel this afternoon:

How I feel this evening:

Today's Anxiety & Stress Analysis

Causes of my anxiety & stress:	How I can change the causes:
1.	1.
2.	2.
3.	3.
4.	4.
5.	5.
6.	6.
7.	7.
8.	8.
9.	9.
10.	10.
11.	11.
12.	12.
13.	13.

Notes

Anxiety & Stress

Date:

How I feel this morning:

How I feel this afternoon:

How I feel this evening:

Today's Anxiety & Stress Analysis

Causes of my anxiety & stress:

How I can change the causes:

Causes of my anxiety & stress:	How I can change the causes:
1.	1.
2.	2.
3.	3.
4.	4.
5.	5.
6.	6.
7.	7.
8.	8.
9.	9.
10.	10.
11.	11.
12.	12.
13.	13.

Notes

Anxiety & Stress

Date:

How I feel this morning:

How I feel this afternoon:

How I feel this evening:

Today's Anxiety & Stress Analysis

Causes of my anxiety & stress:	How I can change the causes:
1.	1.
2.	2.
3.	3.
4.	4.
5.	5.
6.	6.
7.	7.
8.	8.
9.	9.
10.	10.
11.	11.
12.	12.
13.	13.

Notes

Anxiety & Stress

Date:

How I feel this morning:

How I feel this afternoon:

How I feel this evening:

Today's Anxiety & Stress Analysis

Causes of my anxiety & stress:	How I can change the causes:
1.	1.
2.	2.
3.	3.
4.	4.
5.	5.
6.	6.
7.	7.
8.	8.
9.	9.
10.	10.
11.	11.
12.	12.
13.	13.

Notes

Anxiety & Stress

Date:

How I feel this morning:

How I feel this afternoon:

How I feel this evening:

Today's Anxiety & Stress Analysis

Causes of my anxiety & stress:	How I can change the causes:
1.	1.
2.	2.
3.	3.
4.	4.
5.	5.
6.	6.
7.	7.
8.	8.
9.	9.
10.	10.
11.	11.
12.	12.
13.	13.

Notes

Anxiety & Stress

Date:

How I feel this morning:

How I feel this afternoon:

How I feel this evening:

Today's Anxiety & Stress Analysis

Causes of my anxiety & stress:

How I can change the causes:

Causes of my anxiety & stress:	How I can change the causes:
1.	1.
2.	2.
3.	3.
4.	4.
5.	5.
6.	6.
7.	7.
8.	8.
9.	9.
10.	10.
11.	11.
12.	12.
13.	13.

Notes

Anxiety & Stress

Date:

How I feel this morning:

How I feel this afternoon:

How I feel this evening:

Today's Anxiety & Stress Analysis

Causes of my anxiety & stress:	How I can change the causes:
1.	1.
2.	2.
3.	3.
4.	4.
5.	5.
6.	6.
7.	7.
8.	8.
9.	9.
10.	10.
11.	11.
12.	12.
13.	13.

Notes

Anxiety & Stress

Date:

How I feel this morning:

How I feel this afternoon:

How I feel this evening:

Today's Anxiety & Stress Analysis

Causes of my anxiety & stress:	How I can change the causes:
1.	1.
2.	2.
3.	3.
4.	4.
5.	5.
6.	6.
7.	7.
8.	8.
9.	9.
10.	10.
11.	11.
12.	12.
13.	13.

Notes

Anxiety & Stress

Date:

How I feel this morning:

How I feel this afternoon:

How I feel this evening:

Today's Anxiety & Stress Analysis

Causes of my anxiety & stress:	How I can change the causes:
1.	1.
2.	2.
3.	3.
4.	4.
5.	5.
6.	6.
7.	7.
8.	8.
9.	9.
10.	10.
11.	11.
12.	12.
13.	13.

Notes

Anxiety & Stress

Date:

How I feel this morning:

How I feel this afternoon:

How I feel this evening:

Today's Anxiety & Stress Analysis

Causes of my anxiety & stress:	How I can change the causes:
1.	1.
2.	2.
3.	3.
4.	4.
5.	5.
6.	6.
7.	7.
8.	8.
9.	9.
10.	10.
11.	11.
12.	12.
13.	13.

Notes

Anxiety & Stress

Date:

How I feel this morning:

How I feel this afternoon:

How I feel this evening:

Today's Anxiety & Stress Analysis

Causes of my anxiety & stress: | How I can change the causes:

1.

2.

3.

4.

5.

6.

7.

8.

9.

10.

11.

12.

13.

| How I can change the causes:

1.

2.

3.

4.

5.

6.

7.

8.

9.

10.

11.

12.

13.

Notes

Anxiety & Stress

Date:

How I feel this morning:

How I feel this afternoon:

How I feel this evening:

Today's Anxiety & Stress Analysis

Causes of my anxiety & stress:	How I can change the causes:
1.	1.
2.	2.
3.	3.
4.	4.
5.	5.
6.	6.
7.	7.
8.	8.
9.	9.
10.	10.
11.	11.
12.	12.
13.	13.

Notes

Anxiety & Stress

Date:

How I feel this morning:

How I feel this afternoon:

How I feel this evening:

Today's Anxiety & Stress Analysis

Causes of my anxiety & stress:	How I can change the causes:
1.	1.
2.	2.
3.	3.
4.	4.
5.	5.
6.	6.
7.	7.
8.	8.
9.	9.
10.	10.
11.	11.
12.	12.
13.	13.

Notes

Anxiety & Stress

Date:

How I feel this morning:

How I feel this afternoon:

How I feel this evening:

Today's Anxiety & Stress Analysis

Causes of my anxiety & stress:	How I can change the causes:
1.	1.
2.	2.
3.	3.
4.	4.
5.	5.
6.	6.
7.	7.
8.	8.
9.	9.
10.	10.
11.	11.
12.	12.
13.	13.

Notes

Anxiety & Stress

Date:

How I feel this morning:

How I feel this afternoon:

How I feel this evening:

Today's Anxiety & Stress Analysis

Causes of my anxiety & stress:	How I can change the causes:
1.	1.
2.	2.
3.	3.
4.	4.
5.	5.
6.	6.
7.	7.
8.	8.
9.	9.
10.	10.
11.	11.
12.	12.
13.	13.

Notes

Anxiety & Stress

Date:

How I feel this morning:

How I feel this afternoon:

How I feel this evening:

Today's Anxiety & Stress Analysis

Causes of my anxiety & stress:	How I can change the causes:
1.	1.
2.	2.
3.	3.
4.	4.
5.	5.
6.	6.
7.	7.
8.	8.
9.	9.
10.	10.
11.	11.
12.	12.
13.	13.

Notes

Anxiety & Stress

Date:

How I feel this morning:

How I feel this afternoon:

How I feel this evening:

Today's Anxiety & Stress Analysis

Causes of my anxiety & stress:	How I can change the causes:
1.	1.
2.	2.
3.	3.
4.	4.
5.	5.
6.	6.
7.	7.
8.	8.
9.	9.
10.	10.
11.	11.
12.	12.
13.	13.

Notes

Anxiety & Stress

Date:

How I feel this morning:

How I feel this afternoon:

How I feel this evening:

Today's Anxiety & Stress Analysis

Causes of my anxiety & stress:	How I can change the causes:
1.	1.
2.	2.
3.	3.
4.	4.
5.	5.
6.	6.
7.	7.
8.	8.
9.	9.
10.	10.
11.	11.
12.	12.
13.	13.

Notes

Anxiety & Stress

Date:

How I feel this morning:

How I feel this afternoon:

How I feel this evening:

Today's Anxiety & Stress Analysis

Causes of my anxiety & stress:	How I can change the causes:
1.	1.
2.	2.
3.	3.
4.	4.
5.	5.
6.	6.
7.	7.
8.	8.
9.	9.
10.	10.
11.	11.
12.	12.
13.	13.

Notes

Anxiety & Stress

Date:

How I feel this morning:

How I feel this afternoon:

How I feel this evening:

Today's Anxiety & Stress Analysis

Causes of my anxiety & stress:	How I can change the causes:
1.	1.
2.	2.
3.	3.
4.	4.
5.	5.
6.	6.
7.	7.
8.	8.
9.	9.
10.	10.
11.	11.
12.	12.
13.	13.

Notes

www.ingramcontent.com/pod-product-compliance
Lightning Source LLC
Chambersburg PA
CBHW050755160726
48004CB00002B/576